Easing into Practice:

Deep Inquiry Yoga

by

Kim Beyer

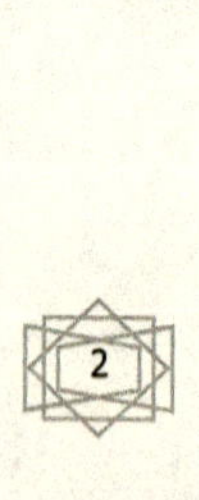

KDP ISBN: 9781790427864

Be sure to visit Kim's blog at

www. vistaandcrossroads.com

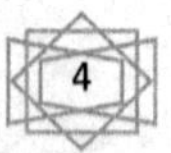

Acknowledgements

It all begins with such a simple question:

"Who am I?"

My thanks to all who engage it,

who hold space as people find their own answers

and who probe the question itself

into Life.

Namaste!

Jaya!

Contents

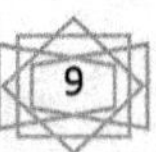

Introducing the Easing into Practice Collection of Books

I came into yoga, and all my spiritual practices for that matter, a bit backward. Long before I tried my first asana, I had read the *Bhagavad Gita, Patanjali's Yoga Sutras,* the *Mahabharata,* the *Ramayana, Shankara,* the works of *Yogananda, Vivekananda,* and *Ramakrishna,* on and on.

Long before I sat down on a meditation cushion, I'd devoured just about every popular book about Buddhist practice and psychology, Neo-pagan traditions, Christian forms of meditation and their contemplative traditions and so forth. I was a sponge, a bibliophile, a perpetual seeker.

It was in graduate school, though, that things did begin to change. I first studied the art of Iaido (meditative drawing techniques of the Japanese sword) then began my gentle exploration of both Hatha Yoga and Qigong and finally completed an entire graduate certificate in holistic health care. Why? Because I was stressed, going through tremendous life changes and found myself at the lonely crossroads where book knowledge could no longer provide a direction forward.

From that seed of a beginning, I committed myself to taking spiritual practice very seriously. I live by a Rule of Life, integrating experiential elements when the deep need of my soul calls for them and sharing what I have learned with others.

I've created this series of books to serve as "first steps" onto the many different paths of spiritual practice. The texts are not exhaustive, but rather, provide an ever-growing pallet of colors for you to explore, adopt and take deeper as you are called. For retreat and adult education professionals, they also become quick reference tools to add depth to your offerings.

Used with my ever-growing companion series of books, *The Easing Into Collection,* (which features the ten great ideas of various world faith traditions, teachers and scripture), the works provide an interlocking introduction to the beauty, complexity and cultural differences and similarities that make spiritual study so engaging and timely. Whether used with small groups or as the springboard to personal study, I believe you'll find both series good companions on your journey.

Namaste and Blessings,

Kim Beyer, MA, CYTh, SD, RM, CHHC, CAFH

www.vistaandcrossroads.com

What is Deep Inquiry Yoga?

There comes a time in every Hatha Yoga practitioner's life when he or she perceives that the physical stretch transitions into an invitation to explore something *more*. We notice that each time we come to the mat, the conditions of the environment, our emotions and thoughts, even the social, financial, and relational energies are completely different, although sometimes on a very subtle level. The truth is, w*e are different each time we practice, and each practice, in turn, changes us.* This is just one facet of the "more" we will be exploring in this book.

I will provide a few suggestions about how to work with this ancient, beautiful and groundless art called Hatha Yoga. *Deep Inquiry Yoga* is a collection of simple practices to apply within the stable and easeful asana to invite the body, breath, mind, intuitive/wisdom self and a taste of joy to simmer together. That simmering cooks you, so you might become an even more fragrant and nourishing dish for yourself and others.

Some of the work between these pages can be done as a small appetizer in a studio classroom or can be used as the central offering of a retreat or during a home meditation time. As always, begin with the practice that is most calling you on a given day—this choice honors the budding intuitive wisdom that is one of the great fruits of a Hatha Yoga practice. That intuitive self is the foundation for a discipline free of studios, teachers and outer lessons and expectations. For each student, there is a shape and sequence for Hatha Yoga—you, and Mystery's grace, will one day be your very best teacher.

Twenty-five years of sharing the techniques in yoga studio, hospital, college and university and community education centers back up these practices. Most are incredibly fresh to me each time I use them on my own mat or teach to others. All are appropriate for beginners. Rest assured, they are time tested friends of mine.

Namaste,

Kim Nunneley, MA, CHHC. CYTh, RM, SD

Practice 1: Heavy and Light

Part of every asana system is learning to turn the movement over to the breath and allow deep and rhythmic inhales and exhales to move and inform the pose. This awareness alerts you to when are not easeful and stable. Perhaps you have stopped breathing fully because the pose is difficult for you right now or your mind has wandered to your grocery shopping list. Injuries happen in Hatha Yoga when your mind disengages from practice. The study of "heavy and light" helps keep you safe as well as creates a dialogue between the body, breath, mind, spirit and your sense of joy, the gross to subtle levels of all embodied beings.

Easeful and *Stable* are the touchstones here. The in-breath tends to create a sense of easefulness and spaciousness, the outbreath a sense of ground and stability. If you are familiar with Patanjali's *Yoga Sutras,* you will recall these two words characterize a proper meditation posture. The same pair of words can be used to inform a mindful Hatha Yoga asana.

Part One:

In a seated or standing position, rest your hands on your belly. Breathing in and out through your nose, tune in to the rise and fall of your breath, feeling the way your hands are *moved by* the flow of breathing. Feel the breath lengthening and then gently compressing the spine.

Part Two:

Allow yourself to feel the inbreath lightening your body. You may imagine you are weightless as the air flows in, and then feel heavy and grounded as you breathe out.

Part Three:

Select a flow of your choice. It can be as easy as a Half Sun Salutation or as challenging as a series of Up Dog to Down Dog Yogic pushups. Mindfully engage with the breath, noticing how the inhale lifts and lightens your experience of the pose creating easefulness, and how the exhale holds and grounds the pose, creating stability. Then, take any held position and again, follow the light to heavy to light sensations within your body. Finally, explore a difficult-for-you asana and notice the effects of your pose on the breath as well as the mind's ability to tune into the heavy and light sensations.

Part Four:

Come to a seated position and consider the following questions. You might want to journal about them or simply check in mentally.

1. How does the practice of light and heavy change the
    way I am able to stay present to my yoga practice?

2. Where, off the mat, would this practice be useful?
    Explain.

3. Did I over-think the heavy and light sensations by
    mentally naming them, or was I able to simply
    experience the effects of the breath?

4. Did I find either heavy or light more enjoyable than
    the other? Why might this occur in myself or
    others?

5. How does Patanjali literally use the terms *easeful* and
    stable in his Yoga Sutras? How might this practice
    also be useful in a formal meditation practice?

Capping Poem:

The fall breeze lifts paper jewels

citrine and ruby and tiger's eye,

all a'swirl with whispers,

sliding over one another,

gazing down at their old rooted tethers

until,

breathless,

they

ground in perfect settings

on porch, and browning grass

or press themselves into

multimedia artforms of stone and sand

beneath

the surface of the sky-mirror lake.

Practice 2: Feeling Prana

As you learn more about Hatha Yoga, you will begin to find yourself face to face with the concept of energy, energy channels, chakras and other subtle (and for the western student, esoteric) elements of being embodied. There are many kinds of pranic energy, and when you get the urge, do a little research to learn more about this subject.

This initial practice is to help students feel prana, using a few moves from what might be thought of as Chinese Yoga or Qigong. Qigong means the work or practice of energy and its repetitive flows may help you tune into the subtle movements of energy in your own body.

Once you've touched this sensation, it becomes much more pronounced in your Hatha Yoga practice. By registering pranic activity, another layer of the Hatha Yoga Deep Inquiry becomes readily available and brings up some interesting questions which we'll explore after the practice.

Part One:

Begin with your feet hip-width apart. Belly button and feet face forward. Next, bend your right knee, and hold an imaginary ball above the knee, about hip-level. Your left hand rests on top of the "ball", your right hand on the bottom. Slowly turn at your waist and shift your weight to the left, rolling the "ball" over. As you come fully into your left knee, your right hand should now be on top. Gently return to the right knee, noticing the left hand now is on top. Continue to move slowly and smoothly, side to side. You can pick a direction to breathe in with and breathe out on the return trip. The breath will help you stay grounded and smooth. Continue for 16 rounds.

Part Two:

Very gradually, begin to decrease the side to side motion, coming at last to a position of stillness with your hands cupping the "ball".

Part Three:

Now draw your hands a bit further apart, then compress just a bit—don't allow your hands to touch! Or roll imaginary cookie dough between your palms. What do you feel? Some folks describe a tingling sensation, others a kind of pressure not unlike the way two magnets push each other apart. A general feeling of warmth may also exist.

Part Four:

Close your eyes and allow yourself to feel your body. Where ever it aches or feels off or cold, rest your hands over this spot without physically touching it. Imagine the place in your body can draw the prana it needs from your hands. You are not pushing it with any sense of will. Allow your mind to stay compassionate and soft. Breathe slowly and mindfully. When you feel ready, return to your standing position without haste. Stand there a moment, in your center, then softly shake your hands as if they were wet. Finish palm to palm, with Namaste hands.

Part Five:

Work through the questions below, either engaging in dialogue in a small group or with your journal:

1. Describe the sensation you experienced in your hands. Have you ever felt something similar in a yoga pose or flow? What do you think you are feeling?

2. How did the aching or "off" part of your body feel when you offered the prana in your hands to that area? What do you think happened?

3. Compare the ideas of nadis (lines of energy in the body) and prana to the Chinese understanding of meridians and chi (qi). Take some time and do a bit of research to gain a deeper appreciation for the similarities and differences between the two energetic systems.

4. How can this practice help you deepen your Hatha Yoga practice? Be specific. Try a few poses and experiment with identifying (or not!) the feeling of subtle energy in the pose.

5. What healing modalities are you familiar with that use a concept of prana or chi? (It's fun to research this a bit as well.) From this brief Inquiry experiment, do you feel differently about those systems than you did before you began this work? Explain.

What is this matrix,

hugging every object,

a candle-blaze in darkness?

What is this tremble,

within the spacious emptiness within my bones,

this pressure

of Nothing against my skin?

Fish that I am,

I have become aware of the water I swim within,

H_2O becoming light,

becoming presence,

becoming a

definition

gone

mute.

Practice 3: Chanting Om with Contraction and Relaxation

Chant is a time-honored practice present in all faiths. Within Bhakti Yoga, the way to union with God through devotion, chant serves as the vehicle to connect practitioners with the Divine. Its effects are systemic—the vibrations are felt within the body, deep and rhythmic breaths calm the central nervous system and strengthen the diaphragm, the mind focuses on a single point, the intuitive self completely opens and is receptive and the sense of joy is given a sweet voice.

Chant can also be an avenue of deep inquiry into the nature and ramifications of contraction and relaxation within the entire body system. It is to this function that we now turn:

Part One:

Take a meditation posture, either on the floor or on a chair. Check in with yourself. Is your back straight, your knees slightly lower than your hips, your hands resting in a comfortable position on your thighs? Sway and wiggle and finally release yourself into a place of ease and stability. Close your eyes.

Part Two:

For this first inquiry, systematically tighten your muscle groups from your feet all the way up into your face and jaw. Bring everything hard and pulled-in—calf, thighs, belly, arms, chest and throat. Draw in your breath through your nose, then chant Om, allowing (as much as is possible) the sound to begin with an "ah" in your belly, then forming the "Oh" in your throat, and finally, at the very end of your breath, intoning "MMM", vibrating especially your hard and soft palate in your mouth as well as your sinuses. Try it two more times, with the body tensed. Pay attention to all the parts of yourself—the body's reaction, the way the breath feels, the state of your mind, any intimations of intuition or a sense of joy. Then release the practice of tension and take in some deep, quiet breaths. Continue breathing until you come into a peaceful, easy rhythm.

Part Three:

For this second inquiry, systematically relax and release your body. You might scan slowly from the feet toward the head, allowing the muscle groups to give into gravity, to expand, to soften. Give your breath permission to effortlessly come and go. Tune into a sense of lightness, buoyancy, and taking up space. When you are established in this deep easefulness, again chant the word OM as you did in the previous inquiry. Complete as many rounds as you wish. In a group, encourage everyone to follow the dictates of their own breathing pace, rather than chanting in a single voice. This will lead to a lovely, multi-layered sound experience. When you are ready, release the practice and return to a soft, abiding presence. Open your eyes.

Part Four:

Let's unpack the experience, either with a small group or in your personal journal:

1. Thinking back to the first inquiry practice, describe, in as much detail as you can recall, what you felt:
   a. In your body
   b. In your breathing rhythm
   c. In the state of your mind
   d. In your intuitive self
   e. In your sense of joy
   f. The overall quality of sound
   g. The overall quality of felt vibration

2. Recalling the second inquiry practice, describe in as much detail as you can recall what you felt:
   a. In your body
   b. In your breathing rhythm
   c. In the state of your mind
   d. In your intuitive self
   e. In your sense of joy
   f. The overall quality of sound
   g. The overall quality of felt vibration

3. Compare the two experiences and the effects of those experiences on the myriad levels of your being. What conclusions did you draw? Did anything surprise you? What are the ramifications for the entire embodied system when you carry tension within it? What are the ramifications for the entire embodied system when you are stable and easeful?

4. For a third inquiry, you may choose to sit at different times of the day, and without any preparation, chant Om or any other vocalization and observe the effects of the practice on your body. Write a bit in your journal about what you discovered.

5. How could this inquiry be used daily in your Hatha Yoga practice? When else might chant be useful for you? How might you add it into your current spiritual practice?

Capping Poem:

Breathe this deviated fifth metatarsal;

Wheezing a little, autumn mold,

typing fingers unfurl,

delicious space between the joints;

Crown rising,

air-head giggle threatening,

pulling the spine along like a string.

What meditation cushion

where, when?

Only Om rising

as belly meets breath meets Mystery

Ah

OH

MMMMMM…

Meet me there,

in the shared silence that follows

and

don't be embarrassed if

you start laughing out loud!

Practice 4: Hand-Dance: Following and Leading

Have you often heard your yoga instructor say, "go at your own pace" or "do what feels right for you" or other such phrases? This practice will show why this is so hard to do in group situations. If you are working alone through this book, you'll need to find someone willing to "inquire" with you for this exercise.

When I teach, folks are often surprised at what comes up for them as they work face to face with another. I also see the ah-ha moments of understanding. Let's see now how you respond to this work!

Part One:

Find a partner and then decide which of you will "lead" first.

Part Two:

With your partner, stand face to face, close enough for your palms to almost touch, but with enough room that you can move with ease. Raise your hands about heart-high. Open your palms and align your own hands with your partner's. Take a moment and tune in to each other's breath. Gaze softly into each other's eyes, a light and yes, sometime humorous contact.

Part Three

The leader then begins to move, while the follower mirrors the movements, attempting to keep their palms lined up with the leader. Notice how you are feeling, physically, mentally, emotionally. Can you identify your breath as well as your partner's? Do you have a sense of intuitive intelligence or joy?

Part Four:

Now, allow the follower to become the leader and again, pay attention to what you are experiencing as you both breathe, gaze and move together.

Part Five:

Come back to your starting position. The first leader will again take over directing the movement, but this time, the idea is to **NOT move or breathe together**. Consciously choose to do your own thing. Maintain eye contact as much as you both are able. Notice what occurs at all the level of your embodied self: body, breath, mind/emotions, intuitive self and your sense of joy.

Part Six:

Change the leadership role again and continue the non-following movement. Keep observing your reactions.

Part Seven:

Come back to the center, hands almost touching the other's at heart level. Create Namaste hands, bowing to each other, to complete the exercise.

Part Eight:

Talk with your partner about what happened, sharing your observations. If you are in a studio environment, you can also pair up with another couple to work through the following questions, open the floor for discussion, or spend time with your journal later.

1. What happened when you and your partner were "linked" by gaze, breath and shared movement? What did you experience at each level of your being?

2. What occurred when you both tried to "not follow"
    the other. How did the experience affect each level
    of your being?

3. What does this experience suggest will happen when
    practicing with others in a yoga class or in any other
    group situation? Do you think the amount of time
    you've practiced yoga could impact your other large
    group experiences? Explain.

4. When in your life have you experienced this "being
    with" or "trying not to be with" sensation? What
    lessons did either situation teach you in the past?

5. How might you create an environment where people
    can honestly pay attention to where *they* are, what
    they need and what *they* are honestly physically
    capable of in any teaching or discussion
    environment? Is this a kind of Yoga in and of itself?
    Explain.

Palm shadowing palm

we giggle together,

even our laughter

riding a synched breath,

wild pony girls,

autumn silver plumes of mirth rising,

lingering,

in the antique insulator-blue sky.

And I?

Forty years later,

Reiki-touching,

still grin,

awash in dim light and spa music,

I catch the scent of damp leaf carpets

and

wisps of cloud-exhales.

Practice 5: Kosha Practice

The koshas are a way to classify our embodied existence on five basic levels of being: the Body, the Breath, the Mind, the Intuitive or Wisdom Self and Joy. It's helpful to think of these labels as strings on an instrument that all vibrate together. For example, if I "pluck" the mind string by watching an irritating news report, there will be a reaction that will be echoed by all the other parts of the system. My emotions and thoughts become agitated, the body tenses, the breath becomes shallow and fast, I pull in my intuitive self to protect it, and my sense of joy becomes a very tiny glimmer within me.

When I turn the program off, I go for a walk with my dog. My body becomes relaxed with the familiar swinging stride, my breath falls into rhythm with my steps, my mind broadens and enjoys the fall foliage, my intuitive-self expands, and I feel joy as a real glow within.

This practice will allow you to clearly access each of the koshas in your Hatha Yoga poses. In the beginning, the work will feel a little cumbersome, but if you continue working with it, like a new asana, it becomes second nature.

Let's give it a try!

Part One:

Choose a stationary pose that is easeful and stable for you—child pose is one such wonderful place to begin. Go into the pose mindfully and with a gentle breath.

Part Two:

Allow yourself to feel all the parts of your body, from the soles of your feet to the top of your head. Bring the back of your body into consciousness as well. Can you feel your pinky toes? Your nose? The back of your ears? Flash on every part of your physical self, not lingering, but simply acknowledging what you can. Then feel the entirety of the physical body. You can try switching rapidly from a small focus (like your thumb) to that more wide-angle appreciation of your whole self.

Part Three:

Still holding the consciousness of body, begin to tune into the breath. What is its texture, its depth, its effects on the physical body? Can you feel it work along the bones, within and around the internal organs? How does the spine react to the breath? Notice, but don't hover or hang on to any one sensation.

Part Four:

Now allow your physical breathing self to feel the presence of thoughts, emotions, memories and even the raw consciousness of the mind. Notice that something in you is watching the movement of the mind.

Part Five:

In this embodied, breathing, conscious form, gently become aware of any intuitive voice—perhaps it is suggesting a small adjustment of some part of the body, or maybe there is a tickle of recognition of your baby-self sleeping in this pose. The "tickle" arises prior to the actual thought, the suggestion to move has a non-verbal "voice" before your mind translates it into word and action. Notice this.

Part Six:

Beneath the body, the breath, the mind, the intuitive self, you may be able to sense a feeling of joy. It's not the confetti in the air sort of feeling, but rather a ground, a base, wholeness. It always reminds me of Julian of Norwich's conviction that "all shall be well, and all shall be well, and all manner of things shall be well."

Part Seven:

Finally, rove back and forth between the body, the breath, the mind, the intuition and sense of joy. You can experiment with holding your breath and observing what happens to all the other koshas. Or bring up a happy memory and then observe its effects on the system that is you. Play for as long as you like and are comfortable in the pose. If you wish, try other poses and flows and notice all five koshas at work.

Part Eight:

In your journal or in a small group or in dyads, consider the following questions:

1. Do you frequently spend more time aware of a single or just a couple kosha(s) in your yoga practice? Why do you think this happens? When you are off the mat, what awareness of the koshas dominate? Why?

2. How might working with all the koshas help you work with the following:
   a. Depression
   b. A creative block
   c. Study
   d. Obsessive thinking
   e. Pain

3. What are the ramifications of the koshas for our Western medical establishment?

4. Did you find it helpful to "compartmentalize" the embodied experience or not? Explain.

5. In yoga classes, how often does your teacher(s)
    access the subtler elements of the fully embodied
    human (intuition, joy)? How might you bring them
    into your practice/teaching at home and off the mat?

Capping Poem:

She flew, headlong, into the clear window,

drunk on fall berries and sunshine.

I cupped her body,

yellow fluff and dazed ink-drop eyes,

her breath outpacing the second hand on my old watch.

I wondered if she could truly see me.

What old fears and memories and instincts

flooded her veins then?

Or perhaps she only intuited warmth and security,

my fingers, a nest, cupping her.

She snuggled for a moment, reviving,

then shivered.

The nest collapsed, and she sprang skyward.

Joy?

I smiled, enough for us both.

Practice 6: Seed and Flower

This is a whimsical practice, great to use with your kids and grandkids, or when you are holding your own Hatha Yoga time with an excessive degree of earnestness. It's a recipe for feeling joy and wonder.

I stumbled across Seed and Flower when I was teaching yoga to children in churches. They remembered the multi-move flow so much better when there was a narrative attached to it, as many folks who teach children are beginning to observe. But this is also true for adults! There is something within us all that resonates with a story.

If you are a teacher, try creating a narrative to accompany complex flows! Or create your own at your home on your mat and share them with others on social media.

Here we go:

Part 1:

Familiarize yourself with *Half-Surya Namaskar*, the half sun salutation.

Part 2:

We add the narrative element with the movement in its story form.

Movement: Namaste hands in front of the heart

Say: "The flower begins with a tiny seed, space within, but also a secret story that allows it to unfold."

Movement: drop hands to the sides and then sweep up until the palms meet overhead.

Say: "The seed feels the sun, warming the darkness, calling it awake."

Movement: Backs of hands meet overhead, then separate, palms pushing out as you hinge at the hips and drop the head toward the floor in a forward fold.

Say: "Roots burst out from the seed, pushing away at the soil."

Movement: Come half-way up, hands just above the knees, spine straight, shoulder blades flat, chin pulled in slightly, gazing at the floor.

Say: "A single stalk rises, a leaf unfurls, lengthens."

Movement: return to the forward fold.

Say: "The roots gather water and food, feeling a strange and wonderful call to climb and bloom."

Movement: rise with big arms, palms up, until the hands meet overhead.

Say: "A glorious flower unfurls itself, its face smiling back at the sun's face."

Movement: return to Namaste hands in front of the heart.

"In the heart of the flower, a seed begins to grow, ready to repeat the story."

Part Three:

Now, select a single word that captures each movement and say the word out loud.

Movement: Namaste hands in front of the heart

Say: "Seed"

Movement: drop hands to the sides and then sweep up until the palms meet overhead.

Say: "Sun"

Movement: Backs of hands meet overhead, then separate, palms pushing out as you hinge at the hips and drop the head toward the floor in a forward fold.

Say: "Roots"

Movement: Come half-way up, hands just above the knees, spine straight, shoulder blades flat, chin pulled in slightly, gazing at the floor.

Say: "Leaf"

Movement: return to the forward fold.

Say: "Roots"

Movement: rise with big arms, palms up, until the hands meet overhead.

Say: "Sunflower"

Movement: return to Namaste hands in front of the heart.

Say: "Seed"

Part Four:

Now, ask yourself to connect with the breath. You may wish to stand and breathe for a few rounds to find your best rhythm and focus. When you are ready:

Movement: Namaste hands in front of the heart

Breathing out, mentally say "seed".

Movement: drop hands to the sides and then sweep up until the palms meet overhead.

Breathe in with the movement, mentally saying "Sun".

Movement: Backs of hands meet overhead, then separate, palms pushing out as you hinge at the hips and drop the head toward the floor in a forward fold.

Breath out with the movement, mentally saying "Roots".

Movement: Come half-way up, hands just above the knees, spine straight, shoulder blades flat, chin pulled in slightly, gazing at the floor.

Breath in with the movement, mentally saying "Leaf".

Movement: return to the forward fold.

Breathe out with the motion, mentally saying: "Roots".

Movement: rise with big arms, palms up, until the hands meet overhead.

Breath in with the motion, mentally saying "Sunflower".

Movement: Return to Namaste Hands in front of the heart.

Breathe out, mentally saying "Seed".

Part Five:

Resume the flow with the silence of your breath, simply feeling the seed, sun, roots, leaf, sunflower and return to the seed, allowing the non-verbal intuitive self to bloom.

Part Six:

When you are ready, cease the flow and stand in Namaste Hands, allowing your whole self to integrate the practice. When you are ready, turn to your neighbor, dialogue as a class or in your journal if you are working with the practice at home and answer some or all these questions:

1. Did the narrative help or hinder your ability to learn this flow? Why do you think this happened? Be concrete.

2. Is it easier to stay connected with the movement when you use the full narrative or when you choose to follow a single word riding the breath? Explain.

3. What other yoga poses or flows can incorporate either a story or a meditative word to help learners retain the memory of the asana?

4. How might you encourage children to create their own "story" about an asana flow? Can you come up with support visuals that might help? Special music? How about a song with the words rather than the spoken version?

5. How did the images of sun, seed, root, leaf, root, sunflower and the final seed change the feel of the flow from the inside, from the level of your intuitive self? It's OK if this didn't happen for you—but talk a bit about the reasons why it didn't.

Capping Poem:

Pony-strides on first-snow path,

suggest

a jaunty tune, me posting in time.

Blue-jay screech

adds an exotic north wood counter-melody.

In the downpour of a violent summer storm,

I hum it yet again,

guiding my blue-eyed mount through puddle and mud,

car horns tooting beyond the show area.

Today, only my dog

his black and white tail waggling

somehow catches the rhythm,

his speckled tongue,

licking it along.

Practice 7: Hard Eyes, Soft Eyes

This is an inquiry that will affect your daily life as much as your yoga practice. We are, by in large, a very focused society. We squint at our cell phones, stare at computer and TV screens, converse eye to eye in coffee houses, or in the relatively small space of our automobiles. Today, we're going to play with the effects of both focused and diffuse awareness, or, as many yoga teachers call it, "hard eyes and soft eyes."

Let's begin:

Part One:

Take up an expansive stationary pose in which you feel both easeful and stable.

Part Two:

Now, harden your eyes. Gaze with intense, unwavering focus at some point in space or on a body part. For example, in Warrior II, you might look along the right arm and then snap in on the middle finger of the right hand. Notice how your entire embodied-self responds—body, breath, mind, intuitive function and sense of joy.

Part Three:

Next, soften your gaze. Try to tune into your peripheral vision, almost as if you could see behind you. Again, notice how the embodied system that is you responds to the wide, diffuse gaze.

Part Four:

Release the pose, come into standing Namaste hands, with eyes closed or gently downcast toward the floor if your balance is iffy.

Part Five:

Take the time to process what this inquiry by working with the following questions:

1. What happened to the embodied system that is you when you attempted the focused gaze? Recount how this felt in:

    a. Your body
    b. Your breath
    c. Your mind
    d. Your intuitive self
    e. Your sense of joy

2. What happened to the embodied system that is you when you switched to the diffuse gaze? Recount how this felt in:

    a. Your body
    b. Your breath
    c. Your mind
    d. Your intuitive self
    e. Your sense of joy

3. If you go through a day with focused awareness as your primary form of attention, what effects do you think it will have on you and others? Or if you go through a day with diffuse awareness as your primary form of attention, what effects will that have on yourself and others? Can you use this practice to choose what kind of attention you bring to the world

and your relationships moment to moment?
Explain.

4. What kind of focus:
    a. helped you feel compassionate and calm?
    b. helped you feel strong and able?
    c. helped you understand the pose at a deeper level?
    d. helped you identify where changes might be made in the pose?
    e. suggested an idea to you that transcended the pose?

5. If you can, recall that moment when you switched from focused (hard eyes) to diffuse (soft eyes) awareness. What happened within the body system at that precise moment? Try to draw a picture or create a poem or dance those impressions to express them to another.

Capping Poem:

Lay your hand on this

the skin of a being

over four hundred years old.

Here, reds and brows and palest greens swirl,

an alcohol ink creation frozen

but more vulnerable than tile.

There, an ant labors skyward,

a small beetle clutched in its pincer-jaws,

threading the canyons of bark.

Step back.

Look up.

Branches flung out and up,

stiff-fingering sky,

tapping neighbor,

bowing as the squirrel tripsy-steps

on a high-wire bough, chittering.

Now ask: which view is tree-ness?

Practice 8: The Gunas

Some yogic philosophical systems believe that all living things are influenced by three basic kinds of energy called the gunas. These energies, in turn, impact the levels of embodied being, a kind of conductor of the symphonic resonance of body, breath, mind, intuitive function and sense of joy occurring within us all the time. (Don't worry, the practice will make this all much clearer and more immediate for you!)

Tamasic energy is like the couch potato, sluggish, indifferent, contractive. Think about how you feel after a huge meal, and you'll have a good beginning grasp of this. Rajasic energy is active, expansive, and sometimes manic. Consider yourself after a strong cup of coffee, and you'll come face to face with rajas. Finally, sattvic energy is centered and balanced, like the glow of watching a sunset, calm and warm and present.

Your yoga practice, too, can reflect and enhance each of these kinds of energetic signatures. Let's experiment with them now:

Part One:

For this exercise, we'll use the very simple pose of *Mountain.* In a standing position, place your feet directly under your hips. Raise your arms overhead, palms separated and facing each other over the crown of your head. Allow yourself to fill out the form with your breath and awareness.

Part Two:

Pretend you really don't want to be on your mat, doing this stupid pose at this ridiculous hour in the morning. In other words, let yourself feel tamasic energy. Notice what happens to your pose at the level of your body, your breath, your mind, your intuitive self and your sense of joy. Perform a forward fold for a few breaths, then return to Mountain.

Part Three:

Now, imagine you are all fired up, eager to show just how amazing you are in this Mountain Pose. People should be clicking picture of you, you are so good! How do you feel now at the level of your body, your breath, your mind, your intuitive self and within your sense of joy as you engage the rajasic energy? When you are ready, drop mindfully in to a forward fold, releasing Rajas. Stay for a few breaths, then gently sweep back up into Mountain.

Part Four:

At last, allow yourself to peacefully abide in the asana. Eyes soft, the pose effortless, breath filling it, mind expansive and calm, little intuitive hints shifting your body, a feeling of joy bubbling but not effusive. This is Sattva. When you are ready, release into a forward fold and stay for a few breaths before returning to standing with Namaste hands.

Part Five:

Let's think about what you observed a bit:

1. Is a pose infused with either tamasic, rajasic or sattvic energy necessarily "better" than the other two energies? Explain.

2. If you watch nature or yourself as you move through the day, can you become aware of tamas, rajas and sattva? How does these energies "fit" into the experience of simply being alive?

3. Do you think it's possible to become "addicted" to any of the three energies? What would the ramifications be for someone habitually tamasic, rajasic or sattvic:

    a. in intimate relationships?
    b. at work?
    c. in their yoga practice?
    d. in their spirituality?
    e. in their political discussions?

4. Do you believe different asana are, by their very nature, either sattvic, rajasic or tamasic? For instance, is the Warrior II pose structured to more quickly become rajasic compared to a child pose's sattvic or even tamasic triggers? How might you work through all three energies in every pose? What do you think it would teach you?

5. Do these energies suggest that there may be a matrix, state, way of being or energy (choose your language) that is beyond or somehow holds all three? Draw, write a poem, dance or find a piece of music to answer this important inquiry.

Capping Poem:

Clumsy, eyes caked with sleep,
he bumbles through the kitchen,
drags himself to the couch
muffin in hand,
blinking.

He reaches for the remote,
slowing leaning forward
as aliens and humans collide
blood spatter 8 AM,
same as coffee.

Commercial on,
he saunters over and leans on the counter,
watching me wash blueberries,
gentle presence,
soft smile.

What is this that holds us?
What
Is?

Practice 9: Tonglen and Welcoming Prayer

How we judge our practice can be source of joy or a source of further suffering. Yes, each of us tends to bring our own brand of discriminating awareness to Hatha Yoga—"is this foot position correct?" "Why aren't I as flexible as he is?" "Come on, you stupid hamstring!" "Wonder what I'll have for breakfast?" "I'm too fat to be doing this." On and on it goes, a constant inner conversation that subtly distances us from the actual experience of our time on the mat.

In this practice, we'll work with a kind and compassionate way to maintain a dialogue with our whole selves as we move through our asanas.

Part One:

Take a seated pose that you find relatively challenging, such as a seated forward fold or a seated runner's fold. Take a moment and breathe and check in with all the parts of yourself.

Part Two:

Identify one place in your body that is particularly tight and place your complete attention there.

Part Three:

As you breathe in, really open to everything you are sensing in this area—the constriction, the heat or cold, the frustration or discomfort. As you breathe out, send this place light, openness, coolness or warmth, an inner smile or other such "gifts". Continue to alternate breathing in the sensations, breathing out compassion and inner gentleness. Come out of the pose when you are ready. If you are doing a right/left pose, repeat this exercise on the other side of your body. Again, come out of the pose and breathe normally, releasing the practice of Tonglen.

Part Four:

Ease into the same pose. When you are settled and breathing comfortably, again focus the mind on a part of the pose that is "talking" to you. This time, as you breathe in, pay attention to the sensations, thoughts and emotions and judgements about the pose. As you breathe out, mentally say "welcome" to those areas. It even helps to allow yourself to try on a soft smile. Continue with the attention-to-welcome cycle for a few breaths. Then allow yourself to come out of the pose mindfully. Again, if you are practicing a pose that has a "right" and a "left" element to it, repeat the practice on the new side. When you are ready, release the practice and the pose, returning to quiet breathing.

Part Five:

You may choose to expand this practice a bit. When you breathe in, you can imagine you are breathing in the discomfort of the pose for every person who has ever experienced the discomfort, as well as the negative or judgmental inner voices. Breathe out the same sense of relief, comfort, compassion and kindness to every person who is experiencing these sensations in a yoga pose. It's interesting to "breathe for each other" in a Hatha Yoga group class.

Part Six:

Take some time to discuss or answer the following questions in your journal:

1. What changes did you observe in the pose as you worked with the breathing practice of Tonglen?

2. Was it more difficult to pay deep attention to the body/mind on the inbreath or to send yourself the compassion and kindness of the outbreath? Why do you suspect this occurs?

3. Was the practice of Welcoming different from Tonglen in any way? Explain.

4. How do you think these practices might be useful for folks just learning yoga? For experienced students?

5. What happened when you practiced Tonglen for others? If you were in a class, what sorts of things "came up" for you and others?

Capping Poem:

Forward fold silence,

the world upside down,

blood rushing in my ears.

Breathing in old rubber-band muscle fibers,

twanging, ancient guitar string flat,

stirrings of

too fat

too old

too lazy

and a dash of

claustrophobia.

Breathing out steady tree trunks,

the sound of a warm wind through willow trees,

the taste of chamomile tea,

the smell of warm apple muffins

the feel of elastic grape vine.

Breathe in,

pay attention.

Breathe out,

a sensual compassion.

Practice 10: Meeting with Your Heart

How do we meet and greet each other, particularly if we don't know each other well? Body language is a fascinating study, one that says a lot about our nonverbalized fears, aggression, and overcompensations. As yogis, part of what we are learning is to bring the whole self into consciousness. Our physical selves speak not only to us, but to the world. This practice will introduce you to a habitual stance that many folks exhibit in our culture and will encourage you to experiment in the world with a new way of being present. The exercises below are for a small group but can be tried with a partner in private.

Part One:

Ask for two volunteers from the group and instruct them to stand about six feet apart. The larger group will observe their interaction. The two should try to be aware of their body language, as well as how their breath, mind, sense of intuition and joy feel in the following encounters.

Part Two:

Allow yourselves to imagine this is a job interview or you are meeting someone you want to impress. You must be competent and strong. You must own this encounter.

Part Three:

Set toward each other and shake hands.

Part Four:

Go back to about six feet apart, close your eyes or lower your eyes and breathe into your belly. Draw your chin in a little and allow attention to drop down into your heart center. Slowly raise your head and look at your partner with soft eyes. Imagine the other is a dear friend.

Part Five:

Step toward each other and again shake hands.

Part Six:

Step back to your starting position, relax and gaze at your partner with soft eyes. Complete the exercise with Namaste hands.

Part Seven:

Sitting in a circle, work through these discussion questions or take up your personal journal and consider what you observed within yourself:

1. When the partners were asked to shake hands like it was a job interview, or you had to "own" the meeting, what did you observe? What did the partners themselves observe?

2. When the duo met from their heart center, what changed from the first encounter? How did the partners feel?

3. Pull up different "meetings" on YouTube. Look at politicians, religious leaders, friends meeting, returning vets, the works. What do you notice about the interactions? What social factors might be affecting the way the different people greet each other?

4. Next time you are in a grocery store, try to greet the register clerk with soft eyes and a sense of being centered in your heart. How did you feel? Was there any reaction from the clerk? Explain.

5. Why do you think we habitually carry the body
   language we do in new situations? How might you
   work with a more mindful approach? What might
   the ramifications be for your life and the lives of
   others?

Parallel play adults,

fingers over the keyboard like claws,

shoulders hunched,

eyes hard,

each line on their faces

blue-screen glare highlighted.

"They."

"Them."

"The Other."

And the media executives smile

radiant dollar signs

and sharp teeth.

Push back.

Wake up now.

Stand in the middle of some grocery store,

watching people hunch,

over thin carts,

eyes not meeting.

Soften.

Weep

for us all.

Practice 11: The Tender Touch

I cringe sometimes when I watch teachers work with students utilizing a "push or pull" method of driving a person into a certain shape in a yoga pose. Yet, sometimes, it's very difficult for a student to be aware of an asana's "backside" when in Downward Facing Dog or a deep twist. We can use leading questions designed to guide a person through a small shift that will stabilize and make the pose more easeful, encouraging their personal Inquiry to self-correct, but sometimes this is not enough. Touch is often the go-to correction at that point. However, we must deeply understand that touch *communicates*—it can blacken a proverbial or not so proverbial eye or say I love you unconditionally.

Let's check out this dynamic out now.

Part One:

Choose a partner. Have one person come into Downward Facing Dog to the best of their ability. The other partner (gently please!) can either pull their hips back or carefully push on the small of the back to encourage the pelvic tilt that creates a strong and beautiful Downward Facing Dog. Use the verbal correction that seems right as well and the touch. The correction-receiving partner should carefully observe their inner reaction on the level of the body, the breath, the mind, intuitive self and sense of joy. The correction-giving partner should do the same! Come out of the pose and both should relax into Reclined Child for six to twelve breaths.

Part Two:

The correction-receiving partner again lifts into Downward Facing Dog. This time the correction-giving partner:

1. asks if a touch is OK to use and waits for a "go ahead." If they are told no, then they act on that no by refraining from touch. This part of the Inquiry is complete.
2. If they get a go-ahead, **use just the soft middle finger of their non-dominant hand** to feather the correction through touch.
3. uses compassionate verbal support here as well.

After a few breaths and observation, return to reclined child.

Part Three:

Change roles and repeat Part One and Part Two above.

Part Four:

Gather the group together or take up journals and answer the questions below:

1. Describe the differences between the two kinds of touch/verbal corrections, being sure to include:

   a. the body.
   b. the breath.
   c. the mind.
   d. the sense of intuition.
   e. the sense of joy.

2. How do you think an experienced Yogi might react to either form of touch? A newbie? Someone who has experienced trauma? A happy go lucky and "huggie" soul? How do you know, without a doubt, how ANY touch will be received? What ramifications does this have for teaching? For you as a student?

3. How do you personally feel about being touched or physically corrected in a yoga class? Are there times when you feel touch is necessary? How does the verbal explanation or asking permission to touch figure into your answer? Explain.

4. Do you think there might be cultural issue that also come into play when we think about touch? Do some research about this topic on the internet or visit with friends from different parts of the world. What did you learn?

5. Are there times when you feel touch is necessary for safety in a yoga class? Explain.

Capping Poem:

When my words fall apart,

shattered into letters,

garbled packages of sound,

into shuddering inhales and exhales,

lay your hand on my shoulder,

soft,

skin on skin.

Somewhere in the shadow of your palm

you hold all languages,

compassion pushing through your fingers

like light.

Practice 12: What Comes Next? Self-Sequencing

Entire books have been written on sequencing and I suspect it sometimes is the single biggest issue that steals a home practice from new Hatha Yoga students. Afraid they will do it "wrong" or injure themselves because of the order they choose to express their poses, they let the mat sit in the corner. But, in most cases, the easiest thing to remember about sequencing is that after a backbend or twist, do a forward fold of some kind. There's no doubt that a well-designed sequence, leading up to a challenging asana can be incredibly beneficial. What I am talking about here is learning to release all the planning and modeling and allow the intuitive self to participate fully in your yoga practice.

Let's explore how this works:

Part One:

Roll out your mat, and then step off it. Place a hand on your belly and the other on your heart, allowing your own touch to calm and center you. As you come into yourself, open to what pose would first like to find expression on your mat. When it is clear, go ahead and begin with that opening asana. Stay or flow for as long as it feels *intuitively* correct.

Part Two:

Come back to stillness, with namaste hands, and allow your intuitive self to suggest what comes next. Notice also what the body, breath, mind and intimations of joy are telling you. This space between the poses or flows may be teeming with not only embodied information, but also an awareness of tamasic, rajasic or sattvic impulses.

If yoga is a great deal about homeostasis, then you'll want to address these gunas—in other words, if you are feeling very slow and groggy, it may be time for a big, heart opening pose or flow. If you are edgy and hard, try a forward fold. If your sattvic, go with it! But watch how this guna rises and falls as well. But be aware that your intuition may over-ride this logic. Trust yourself.

When you are ready, take the next pose that your entire embodied self knows is right for you.

Part Three:

Continue to alternate a pose or flow with a time of stillness and listening for what comes next.

Part Four:

Finish with at least ten minutes in Corpse Pose (Savasana) and allow yourself to accept the fruits of your practice.

Part Five:

Take up your journal or get face to face with a partner and play with the questions below:

1. How did this practice affect:

    a. Your sense of your body?
    b. Your breath?
    c. Your mind?
    d. Your sense of intuition
    e. Your awareness of internal joy?

2. Describe how it felt to listen deeply before moving into the next flow or asana. In other words, were you unsure? Elated? Bored? Why?

3. How might you incorporate this intuitive practice if you are teaching a yoga class? For example, with an experienced group of yogis, towards the end of the class, I'll often just ask them to take the next pose that feels natural to them. What other information will need to enter the picture to help you paint a lovely experience? What resources could new students use to more deeply explore "what comes next"? Be creative!

4. How might you deal with the isolation that sometimes is felt during a home practice? What wisdom can you impart or make use of?

5. How do you think the practice of listening to yourself might affect the way you go through the world "off your mat"?

Capping Poem:

Mourning practice-

even the sky is gray,

sound-canceling clouds

padding birdcalls

and leaf-whisked grass.

The lake mirrors the heavens,

dimming the far shore

and oozing the sand.

I stand on my mat,

hands pressed in Namaste,

waiting.

I could spring into

sun salutations and warrior poses,

but

just now

I let myself

fold toward the earth

and all the world

holds me.

Practice 13: Wiggling In

I am a big proponent of wiggly yoga. In a way, it's a form of deep listening on all the channels of yourself, along with a dose of hypothesis and experimentation. Rather than forcing yourself into a perfect pose and holding it like a dismount from the bars at a gymnastics meet, this form of entry into a stationary pose is fluid, playful and internally paced. It allows you to find the edge of what you want to do, testing each side of it, weighing the asana from within.

Fewer injuries, especially for young and new practitioners, is just one of the benefits of this sort of inquiry. Let's check it out:

Part One:

Choose a seated stationary pose. Set up the asana with very little sensation feeding back to you. For instance, if you are trying on a seated twist, move to the very first tickle of resistance. Breathe into that sensation with all the parts of yourself.

Part Two:

Gently deepen the pose, riding the first half of the breath cycle, then release to the level of beginning sensation again. So, if you are trying that seated twist, you would exhale a little deeper into the twist, inhale and return to your starting point. Do NOT move into any kind of pain or strain. Observing a broken rhythm of the breath or a sense of "flight or fight" in your mind or body are just two signals that you're going too far, too fast. Adjust and flash on a sense of patience, non-harming and compassion for yourself.

Part Three:

You can absolutely shift, adjust, play and roll pockets of tension you encounter as you move in and out of the pose. This is the "wiggly bit" and it often feels like a lovely massage! Notice if each deepening changes something about the pose. Also, carefully observe how the body, breath, mind, sense of intuition and joy respond to your technique.

Part Four:

When you are satisfied you have found the best pose for yourself today, hold and breathe. Again, notice all the effects of the experiment on your embodied self. If you are practicing a two-sided, left-right asana, go to the other side and repeat the inquiry. It may prove very interesting—we are not the same on the left and right, and this will often become obvious with this technique. Don't judge! Practice ahimsa—non-harming. Just observe.

Part Five:

You may need to do a counter pose if you chose a twist or backbend. Practice this technique with the counterpose. Then, sit quietly for a few breaths, observing the effects of the entire inquiry.

Part Six:

Dialogue or journal with the following questions:

1. How did this technique differ from how you usually engage with a yoga posture?

2. What was the effect of this inquiry on your:

    a. Body?
    b. Breath?
    c. Mind?

d. Sense of intuition?

e. Sense of joy?

3. What do you need to be mindful of if you teach this form of entering a Hatha Yoga asana?

4. As a student, how can you best allow yourself to use this technique in a class? At home?

5. What are the benefits and drawbacks of this inquiry? Can you think of where a gradual, get your toes wet slowly approach is also important in relationships or in your work? Be concrete.

In the sunlight, he drops into

a canine downward facing dog,

his white and black patches shimmering,

tail lengthening the stretch,

paws massaging the wood floor,

pelvis shifts a bit,

coat shivering in delight,

eyes focused on some internal yumminess.

He lets it all go,

drops asana practice with a changing-gears shake,

then

the laughing, lolling tongue tastes the air

for the hint of his well-toothed bone

surly hiding under a soft cushion.

I bow to the Master of the pose.

Practice 14: Rehearsal Effect

I often call this practice 4, 3, 2, 1. It gets its name from the sports world where it means to slowly and carefully learn to coordinate the body, gradually adding speed, precision or smooth movement as muscle memory (and as we Yogis know, so much more!) to shift the learner from study mode to spontaneity. Used with flows of all kinds, it's a delightful way to teach a new vinyasa or simply create more attention to both the breath and linked poses themselves. On cold Michigan mornings, it has proven to be a warmth-generating and yet mindful technique to awaken the whole-body complex. New students tend to appreciate this approach because it gives them time to really feel the transitions between each asana, as well as how the breath functions to move the vinyasa along. The greatest impact may be at the level of the mind. Observe what happens as you try on this exercise.

Part 1:

We'll work with whatever form of the sun salutation you are familiar with. (However, it works just as well with Moon Salutations, and other variants. Feel free to adapt, honoring your intuitive self.) The first part of the practice I name "the practice of fours".

1. From Namaste Hands, inhale (1) up into mountain or a soft standing backbend. Stay for three more inhales, then,
2. exhale into the forward fold. Stay for three more exhales, then
3. inhale into jack-knife. Stay for three more inhales, then
4. exhale forward fold, staying for three more exhales, then

5. inhale standing runner right, staying for three more inhales, then

6. exhale plank, staying for three more exhales, then

7. inhale *chaturanga dandasana* three more inhales, then

8. exhale downward facing dog, staying for three more exhales, then

9. inhale upward facing dog, staying for three more inhales, then

10. exhale downward facing dog, staying for three more exhales, then

11. inhale standing runners stretch left, staying for three more inhales, then

12. exhale standing forward fold, staying for three more exhales, then

13. inhale jack-knife, staying for three more inhales, then

14. exhale standing forward fold, staying for three more exhales, then

15. inhale to mountain or gentle backbend, staying for three more inhales, then

16. exhale namaste hands, accepting the fruits of the practice.

Part 2:

Repeat the above, staying with each discrete pose for a 3-count inhale or exhale. The breath moving you into the asana is always "one", then stay for X-more. So, you inhale a pose (one), stay for two more inhales for a total of three. This is the practice of threes.

Part 3:

Repeat the above, this time using the practice of twos. The first half-breath moves you into the pose, stay for the second, then transition. This is the practice of twos.

Part 4:

Now, complete the usual vinyasa, riding the breath (the practice of one). When you have completed several normal vinyasa sequences, release the practice mindfully.

Part 5:

In group discussion or with your journal, consider the following questions:

1. How did your body, breath, mind, intuitive self and sense of joy react to the inquiry at each stage, from practice of fours to the normal flow? Did you observe any impatience? A deeper sense of where you were in space and the importance of your breath? Describe and explain!

2. What other sports make use of a rehearsal effect? Can you give examples?

3. Where in your life can you break down a skill, slowing a process down to learn it well, then put it all back together again? Come up with three separate instances where this might work.

4. How could the three gunas possibly affect this inquiry?

5. Would you expect a class to be able to do this practice all together, lock step? Is this true of all vinyasa? Why? How would you teach this in a studio setting?

Feather the fingers over the holes,

breathe the sequence again,

finding this trilled tongue,

that micro-roll of muscle,

creating a breezy path from

heart to instrument to Mystery.

In my sleepy evenings,

the practice continues,

wiggling digits against his ribs,

playing nerve endings from joy to union.

Perhaps all this life is rehearsal,

reverberating within.

Practice 15: What Color Arises?

One of the most interesting discernment programs I took part in about ten years ago used a technique to move from the thought-locked left-brain to the creative right-brain. When faced with two different paths, I was asked a simple question: what kind of dog would path A suggest? What kind of dog would path B hint at? I almost laughed aloud—except, it worked! Path A took the form of a Doberman, complete with a studded black leather collar. Path B appeared in the form of a Golden Retriever, her long tail fanning the air. Either path was "doable", but one definitely carried the energy of kindness and warmth.

In this inquiry we'll be doing a similar sort of thing, allowing the pose to be processed by our intuition and then further chewed on by the symbol-utilizing portion of our mind. Rather than discerning between two or more courses of action, we'll get a new glimpse at how a given pose is affecting our whole selves.

This practice works well individually and as a class—it's fun to compare the similarities and differences that arise and makes for great conversations about how we assign meaning to something as ephemeral as color. It's also possible to do this Inquiry using different senses. For instance, you can ask, "how does this asana smell?" "What food is this like?" "What fabric or texture comes to mind in this pose?" "What piece of music or instrument comes to mind?" Have fun!

Part One:

Begin with a pose that is comfortable for you. Breathe into it, filling it out and allowing yourself to become fully present to all aspects of the asana—body, breath, mind, intuitive self and a glimmer of joy. Then ask yourself, "what color is this pose?" Wait until your intuitive-self responds with an answer that your mind can hold and remember. Release the practice, and when you are ready, jot the name of the asana and the color down in your journal.

Part Two:

Repeat with other poses, at least ten to fifteen, gradually moving on to asanas that are challenging for you. After each, take the time to note the name and color that arose for you in your journal.

Part Three:

Finish your inquiry with some time in relaxation pose.

Part Four:

With your journal, list the different colors you used and then describe what each color means for you. This is wildly individualist on some level, and on others, it's partially determined by your society! For instance, broadly speaking, white is the color of funerals and renunciates in India, while red is the color of purity. It's why you don't see brides in white in India! Consider another sense: while lavender as a scent is touted to relax and calm folks, people in the late 1800s used lavender to cover the scent of death during funerals, and so would not have calmed most folks of that era, but rather, reminded them of loss and grief.

If you decided to work with another sense, simply do the same kind of analysis—what does this sound mean to you? What does this scent bring up for you? And so on.

Part Five:

When you have identified how you respond to colors, assign your response to the asana list you created during practice. For instance, your list may look something like this:

Half-Moon Pose

Color: aspen leaf yellow

My Intuitive Definition: expansive, glowing from within. Some hints of time passing.

Child Pose

Color: foggy gray

My Intuitive Definition: tamasic, a little sad, unenthused today

Or

Half-Moon Pose

Color: scent of green tea

My Intuitive Definition: cool, bright, aware

Child Pose

Scent: home baked bread

My Intuitive Definition: calming, comforting, safe

Part Six:

Now, take the time to consider the following questions through group dialogue or in your journal:

1. Looking at your list, do you notice certain families of poses share a similar color spectrum? If you were using a different sense, do certain families of poses trigger similar responses? For instance, do forward folds of all kinds elicit a similar symbolic or intuitive response? Explain.

2. Were you able to see any aversion or attraction to certain families of poses? To one or two individual poses? Why do you think this is occurring?

3. Can you identify the linking of a certain sense with a specific asana with your social norms? In other words, perhaps in a meditative pose, a "navel gazing" or tamasic negative response from parts of our society influenced the way the pose was perceived for you. When or from whom do you think this message came from? Be as specific as you can.

4. How could assigning color or another sense to a pose be used in the creation of poetry, art, music, and so forth? Explain or demonstrate!

5. How was this inquiry useful to you personally? What did you learn about your practice as a whole?

Capping Poem:

Crane pose white chocolate melts

over a squat-muffin,

rising to form a

tomato soup steam mountain,

flowing exuberant curry backbend,

chased by a

cherry dessert wine

forward fold.

How can I not be fed?

Burp.

Practice 16: Music and Hatha Yoga

Step into most Hatha Yoga classes and you will find, or rather *hear*, what? Usually music! Here is the question, though: what effect does music have on your yoga practice and why is it used almost universally in studio settings? The answers you discover may surprise you because music, like color, lighting, scents, images, and so on speaks to a very subtle part of you. These are the tools of the propagandist as well as the very lifeblood of aesthetics, art and entertainment of all kind. Our work here is to becomes aware of the effects of just one part of the environment where we practice Hatha Yoga.

Part of Yoga is the cultivation of deep inquiry, of discerning how our inner embodied self interfaces and dances with our environment. It's about awakening, within and without, to more and more subtle messages, intuitions, compassion and this thing we call reality.

So, lets tune in to how music functions in a Yoga practice.

Part One:

Pick out four distinctly different kinds of music, with two or more songs from each genre you've decided upon. You might select something calm and instrumental, a strong classical music piece, a pop song you like, and then something like Polka, Blue Grass or Chinese classical music. Mix it up; don't stay with music you love and know.

Part Two:

Create for yourself a short ten-minute or so yoga routine. You'll be using the same routine with each of the four kinds of music you have selected.

Part Three:

Play your first set of songs, performing the routine you've designed. Immediately after the routine and music have ended, jot down some notes for yourself. It may help to organize the notes in the following way:

1. What did I feel in my body?
2. What did I notice about my breath?
3. How did my mind function during this experience? What emotions popped up? Judgments or appreciation? Memories?
4. What nudges of intuition came up?
5. Could I feel the textures of joy within me?

After you've answered the questions, simply sit and allow yourself, in silence, to return to a mindful and present attitude within and without.

Part Four:

Work through all four genres of music, taking careful notes after each. Always "clean your palate" with a brief meditation time.

Part Five:

In large or small group dialogue or with your journal, consider the following questions:

1. As you look over your notes, what kinds of music encouraged and supported you in your practice? How do you know?

2. What kinds of music made your practice more difficult?

3. Do you think music is perceived universally the same? How might this affect a Hatha Yoga class?

4. Why do you think music is used so often in Yoga classes? Come up with several reasons why this a useful tool as well as several reasons why it may be best to turn the music off. How will you choose to practice and teach and why?

5. When we consider the scientific fact that if you study with X kind of music, your recall of study information will be much greater if you are again listening to X kind of music, how does this impact the ability of students to access asana in their memories? What are the positive and negative ramifications of this for the Hatha Yoga practitioner? How can this aspect be used to "brand" specific kinds of Hatha Yoga?

Fabric swish,

the thump on my foot hitting the mat,

off-balanced lunge exasperation brass,

the thin high sigh of my breath,

beginning again,

re-finding the progression of muscle notation

counterpoint birdsong and

snow crystals against the window interlude.

Practice 17: Receiving Your Practice

When you're ready to turn inward and really open to your
Hatha Yoga poses, this is the inquiry to tap. It's particularly
lovely when you are anxious or scattered (what sometimes is
called Vata derangement). Keep a light blanket nearby to
use in Savasana (Relaxation or Corpse Pose) if your studio
or practice space is chilly or if you need a little extra
"holding". Don't expect to go through more than six to ten
poses in an hour session and be sure to choose poses that
work through the range of openings. I've included a sample
below but use your intuition to pick what you need on a
given day.

Part One:

Assemble your mat and blanket and eye pillow if you use it.
Choose silence to work with rather than music today. Yes,
please do experiment with music added to this inquiry at
another time!

Part Two:

Here is a suggested list of poses. It's helpful to keep the list
next to you if you choose to use it. You can also just
intuitively move from pose to pose—your practice, your
choice!

1. Half Sun Salutation
2. Warrior 1, right and left
3. Wide Angle Downward Facing Dog
4. Triangle Pose **or** Side Angle Pose
5. Cat/Cow Flow
6. Cobra
7. Seated Forward Fold
8. Seated Twist
9. Recline Child Pose

Part Three:

Begin in Relaxation pose for about five minutes. If you are jittery, try resting your hands on your belly or cover yourself with your blanket. When the time is up, mindfully ease yourself into the first pose. Stay focused and aware of every move, of the breath, of the mind, your sense of intuition and joy. Stay for at least six to twelve breaths.

Part Four:

Return to Relaxation Pose, receiving your practice. Carefully observe the echoes of the previous pose in your body and allow yourself to be particularly mindful of the transition from the asana to the Relaxation Pose. Stay in Savasana for at least three to five minutes.

Part Five:

Work your way through each of the asana on the list, pausing for the Savasana period between each pose.

Part Six:

Stay in the last Relaxation Pose for ten to fifteen minutes, more if you feel you can stay open, conscious and present.

Part Seven:

Rise to sitting meditation posture or a chair if necessary. Intone three Oms to transition before working with the questions below:

1. What did you notice most about this inquiry? Be specific.

2. Did you chafe at only working through a few asanas? Where do you think this emotion came from? If you sank into the inquiry like a

proverbial duck to water, why do you think this occurred?

3. Were you more conscious of your transitions between asana? Explain.

4. Was settling into Savasana difficult at first? Did it become easier? How did the final Relaxation Pose feel compared to other times you've settled into that asana?

5. Describe the state of your mind at the end of this practice. What does your intuition tell you about why you are feeling this way?

Capping Poem:

Snow tornado in lamplight,

shot through with reds, yellows, surly browns,

fall and winter contending,

howling,

teenage boys shoving

at tree and lake and bundled diners.

Morning waves a pink and blue truce flag,

hint of snow on the rooftops,

grass and flowers open-armed for the drips,

a handful of damp leaves

arrayed in messy curves

by the porch door.

Practice 18: Moving Prayer

I am, by nature, an "in my head" kind of woman. And obsessive thoughts, twanging my entire embodied system do occur, more often than I like to admit. In a sense, such thoughts can become mantras of the negative. If this sounds familiar to you, this inquiry is designed to use that unfortunate energy to your advantage. You can utilize this repetitive nature of thought to turn your asana practice into a time of mental prayer as well.

Let's observe how this works:

Part 1:

Select a few words or phrases that have meaning to you. They may be affirmations, they may be lines from the Bible, the Qur'an, the Bhagavad Gita or literature. They may be lines from a song you love. The important thing is to select something that resonates with your heart.

For example, I often use:

> Thy Will be Done
>
> Om Shanti Om (Om Peace Om)
>
> I am enough.
>
> My all beings be free of suffering.

You can also jot down ten or fifteen such phrases and place them in a bowl, selecting one at random each day.

An alternative to actual words is flashing on an image—instead of a phrase, bring a specific image to mind during the practice below, such as a sunrise, an up-close flower portrait or an icon.

Part Two:

Carefully notice the state of your body, breath, mind, sense of intuition and joy before you begin. As you work through your asana practice, simply say your word or phrase on the out-breath and allow yourself to inhale silence and awareness of your pose. It's best to do this work without music or other auditory distractions. If you are teaching this inquiry to a class, be sure to keep instruction about the poses to a bare minimum. You can certainly "try the inquiry on" with just a few poses during your class time.

Part Three:

During Savasana, release your words and receive your practice in silence.

Part Four:

In groups or with your journal, play with the following questions:

1. Did the state of your embodied-self shift during this inquiry? How did it affect:

    a. Your body?
    b. Your breath?
    c. Your mind and emotions?
    d. Your sense of intuition?
    e. Your sense of joy?

2. Did the practice help or distance you from your experience of each individual pose? Why do you think this happened?

3. Could this be a useful technique to use "on the spot" and off the mat? Explain.

4. Do you believe "we become what we think"? How might this philosophy impact this inquiry?

5. How could you tweak this practice to use with children or teenagers? How could it be used as "medicine" after surgery or illness? Explain.

Capping Poem:

Roll the words mindfully,

thought-finger notes,

paced in time with step,

with breath,

with breeze-chilled blinks.

Long after the sound packages

dissipate,

soaking cement and rust-edged flowers and gray clouds,

mind folds gleam--

prepared canvas,

dusted keyboard,

expectant.

Practice 19: Pass the Pose Storytelling

Sometimes, it's important to bring joy to the fore-front during a yoga class. So often, we approach Hatha Yoga with a rajasic, do or die, feel the burn sort of attitude. Very earnest. Very serious. And sometimes, this is lovely. But life is made up of textures—happiness, grief, rage, joy, peace and disturbances. When we can allow these rivers to flow within the practice of Hatha Yoga, we are better able to face reality off the mat.

I have used this technique with teens, in a class right after a long, hard private school day. Sometimes the story was light and funny but other times, they told a tale that would make tears come to the eyes of most focused yogi or yogini. As a teacher, be prepared to hold space and allow, allow, allow. You direct the flow of the inquiry, but not the content. It's an interesting way to step out of controlling a classroom situation and into intuitive space.

Let's create our story:

Part One:

Carefully explain the following directions to the class. (You'll find your student will need a basic understanding of pose terminology. I've sometimes put up a chart of about fifteen possible poses to choose from to help here.) This technique can be used with as few as two people, who simply pass the pose to each other in succession. It's helpful to remind the students to always pick a pose from the forward fold family after a backbend or twisting form.

The leader can designate how the story flows from person to person. You can work down rows, around the circle or whatever works best for the space, or the teacher can simply move physically near the next person to signal who goes next. Try to design a way to pass the story that doesn't require anyone to remember what specific number they are. People tend to forget during the inquiry!

Part Two:

The leader or volunteer begins the story with a pose of their choice. For example, he or she might say:

"The old dog stretched in the sunlight." They then take up Downward Facing Dog, and the class follows.

The next person might say, "When someone knocked at the door, he growled like a lion," moving into lion pose and roaring out loud.

The following participant chimes in, "When the knocking stopped, he yawned, rolled on his back, sticking his legs straight up into the air!" And then perform Reclined Plank Pose.

Keep passing the story as long as you wish! It's a nice interlude to do this for just part of a yoga class when students are dull, spacey or unfocused. Remember, sometimes it takes a bit to shift from asana to the story line—encourage folks to take their time! It's all part of the fun.

Part Three:

Find a way to release the story. You might applaud, have everyone take a bow, and so forth. Trust the energy in the room. Sometimes it all falls apart in fits of laughter, with hugs all around. Sometimes it peters out with embarrassed giggles. It's all perfectly natural and OK.

Part Four:

Pair off into dyads or work with your journal and consider the following questions:

1. How did the experience impact

    a. your body?
    b. your breath?
    c. your mind?
    d. your sense of intuition?
    e. your sense of joy?

2. What resistance(s) or playfulness did you experience
    during this exercise? Why do you think this
    occurred? Are there other times in your life when a
    similar reaction popped up? Explain.

3. How does the construction of a Hatha Yoga story
    affect the way you view folks in your class? Did it
    change how you viewed your instructor?

4. What part does a sense of play have in your own life
    off the mat?

5. Do you think other practices like Laughter Yoga,
    Baby Goat Yoga, Bring Your Pooch to Class Yoga,
    Couples or Partner Yoga and Disco Yoga have a
    place in the Hatha Yoga tradition? Why do you
    think these practices crop up from time to time?
    Explain.

Telephone game,

mouth-to-ear whispers,

the story flowing around the circle,

its wisp-body shifting,

leaning jean,

conspirator watch,

pink lip-gloss flashing

cowboy boot tapping

evolving, devolving

scattered puzzle pieces,

petals picked from the daisy head,

all loosed

with giggles.

Practice 20: Who Are You?

This question is the central inquiry of Jnana Yoga, the way to union that uses the mind to transcend the mind. It's particularly poignant for Western Hatha Yoga practitioners. I recall a time when the gym I worked for wanted promotional pictures of all its Yoga instructors. The gal I was pair with was indignant that I didn't want to do headstands on an autumn park bench. In my mind, I was a bit resistant to pictures at all—my students by and large were over sixty years old, thoughtful and kind and we functioned as a community rather than a hierarchy. I didn't want to be their posterchild. Besides that, I've only done a bonified headstand maybe three times in my entire career. A severe old neck injury contraindicates that kind of inversion, unless I use a contraption to keep any pressure off the top of my head.

The impasse really came down to who we thought we were—instructors or facilitators, the playful and strong and outlandish Yogini or the contemplative, retiring, and gentle yogini. It was tinged with how our students viewed us, how we "thought" the public might interpret us and Hatha Yoga, on and on.

In the end, my picture was a simple and joyful Warrior I, hers was an inversion on a park bench. Which was really a good portrait of a modern Hatha Yoga instructor? Probably both. Maybe neither.

Let's try to answer this question now:

Part One:

Before your Hatha Yoga practice, take out your journal or make sure everyone has a sheet of paper and a writing instrument. Share with your class that they should answer this one question as quickly and with as many examples as they can: Who Am I?

> I am…a mother

> I am…a wife

> I am…Kim

> I am…poet

> I am a…dog lover

> I am…me

Try to create at least 25 separate lines, and the more the better.

Part Two:

When everyone has completed the task to the best of their ability, ask your class to

1. Cross out any sentence that is a role. For instance, wife, social worker, bank manager, yogi or yogini, mother, poet are all roles. Tell them they are not their ROLES.

2. Cross out any sentence that is a given name. For instance, I would cross of the name "Kim" above. Tell them they are not simply their NAMES.

3. Cross out any sentence that is a specific gender, such as woman, man, teenage girl, and so on. Tell them they are not their GENDERS.

4. Cross off any sentence that is judgmental, such as angry, happy, lighthearted, grumpy, well-liked, disliked and so on. Tell them they are not passing JUDGMENTS.

5. Cross off any sentence that is symbolic, such as child of God, sinner, spiritual being having a human life, or anything like these examples. Tell them they are not SYMBOLS.

6. Cross off any sentence that serves as a physical or mental label, such as asthmatic, diabetic, depressed individual, and so on. Tell them they are not LABELS.

7. Cross off any sentences referring to age, race, national affiliations or academic titles. For instance, they'd delete I am fifty, I am ¼ Native American, I am a Canadian, I am a Ph.D. candidate. Tell them you are not your AGE, RACE, NATIONALITY or TITLES.

8. When you are done, have folks call out what is left on their list, and see if they are some subset of the above. For instance, I sometimes hear the very earnest answer "I AM"! But expressed in this way, those are just words, an imprecise symbolic representation based on a collection of ideas. That not who the person is!

9. Finally, when all the options have fallen silent, ask again, "Who am I? Who are You?"

Part Three: After a brief meditation period, begin your Hatha Yoga class, asking that people silently hold the question "Who am I?" when they are breathing in stable and easeful poses. They may also use this question in Relaxation Pose, allowing it to dissolve into pure awareness.

Part Four:

After Savasana, pose the following questions:

1. What did you learn from this inquiry?

2. Did you experience a sense of groundlessness?
    Panic? Wonder? Explore why a very strong
    emotional response to the inquiry might have
    occurred.

3. How did this important question of "who am I" affect
    your Hatha Yoga practice?

4. Is it possible to express who you are using language?
    Music? Visual arts? What other way can you BE
    "who am I?" Show a partner or the class if you come
    up with something! Is this who you are?

5. How do you live into "Who am I?" off the mat?

I am

popcorn chased with M & M's,

the farewell smell of flowers edged with frost,

the sound of a dog's toenails skating wood floors,

the towering blue spruce leaning away from passing cars,

the cotton and curry feel of a sari quilt from India,

a memory of my grandmother's blue canning jar,

an urge to take up wood carving,

a shudder of migrating sadness,

a lip-tickling tongue twister,

I am.

Don't read on. Be here with me!

Who better?...

Practice 21: Intercessory Prayer Practice

In times of grief or trauma that touch us all, we often want to do SOMETHING. But that isn't always possible. The earthquake that shattered Indonesia, the ambulance that rushed by you, lights flashing during the morning rush hour, the teenager hunched over after his first girlfriend brushed him off may all loom heavier than any action or word can cure.

These events are liminal times, doorway and garden gate passages of life. And while yes, I am very supportive of any active, helping and concrete impulse that arises within you, I would also like to suggest this following inquiry as a form *contemplative* "doing".

Part One:

Name the situation you are engage with, whether some far-reaching calamity like a category five hurricane or something completely personal like an illness or rejection. Say it out-loud, then hold its name in silence for three to five minutes.

Part Two:

Place the name of the person or place experiencing the tragedy in your heart. You certainly can name yourself, by the way. As the work of this Inquiry progresses, you don't have to intone or mentally keep repeating the name or the situation here. Just let its presence gently surface time to time in your consciousness and intention. Proceed with your asana practice, framing each pose with a touchback of Namaste hands and tuning into the situation again and again. Try not to "fix" anything. Merely hold all the aspects of the issue, the people involved, the land or whatever else befriends your attention.

Part Three:

Totally release your focused attention on the issue during Savasana—as some would say, "give it to God" or "Let it Be." Sometimes, it helps to breathe an "Amen" or "Om Shanti Om" or the like before letting go into relaxation pose to create a sense of completion or fulfilled intention.

Part Four:

When you are ready, take up your journal, meet in dyads or in a group discussion and consider the following questions:

1. How did you respond to this practice on the level of

    a. your body?
    b. your breath?
    c. your Mind?
    d. your intuitive self?
    e. your sense of joy?

2. Do you feel such practice has efficacy for all personal and non-personal elements and players involved in the situation? Why or why not?

3. What do you think the purpose of intercessory prayer is for the human being, across all religious and racial affiliations? Is there some universal need for this kind of attention? Explain.

4. Did you balk at the name of this Inquiry? What could you name it that would feel more comfortable to you? In your own opinion, do you think this kind of practice requires the presence of a deity, so you might be "heard"? Explain.

5. If you practiced in a group setting, was there a different tone to the entire Hatha Yoga sequence of

poses and rest? Can you describe it? What are the
ramifications of what you observed?

Writing workshop,

Eight AM spring birdsong.

He walked us through his daughter's rape

and murder

and resting place beneath some gnarled apple tree

just pushing its sap into tentative blooms.

Coffee sits poorly, sloshing against sugar-coated donut
holes,

pen rolling between thumb and pointer finger,

its red tip shying away from the print,

prefers to be held

but not too tightly.

Practice 22: Drawing it Out

The delight of a Hatha Yoga practice is working not only with our inside experience of the pose but the real beauty of poses when viewed from outside. Breathtaking photography and painting and sculptures, as well as music, poetry and more have probably made their way into your consciousness via social media, mainstream media, art galleries, and so on.

This Inquiry is another playful one, but with a serious intent behind it. What we can observe and then create from, we must know deeply. This exercise requires a partner, a class or you can make do with a big mirror!

Let's begin.

Part One:

Assemble colors or pencil and ink drawing material, and sketch pads. I've even played with pastel, water color, crayon, acrylic and alcohol inks, but make sure you've placed plastic around to protect your floor or your yoga mat!

Part Two:

If you are working with a class, divide the group into folks who will demonstrate poses and another that observes, then switch roles immediately after the first asana has been completed. Now the other half will watch the asana each person selects.

Students should choose a pose that they'd like to explore in more detail, and if they are daring, encourage them to pick one they don't much care for. Ask them to move in and out of the pose mindfully, observing on all the levels of their being.

The observation group is not looking for technical perfection! Rather, request participants to allow images, smells, sound, tastes, textures to arise as they observe one pose in the group. (In a class, there may be many asanas to choose from!)

Part Three:

After both sides have had a chance to both observe their chosen pose from within and without, ask them to use the art materials to respond to the pose they observed. It could be a poem, a wash of colors without any form, a black and white sketch, on and on. There is no one "right" response.

Part Four:

In dyads or with your journal, play with the following questions:

1. Discuss what came up for you as you expressed the asana on paper. Your conversation may range from your fear of artistic work to the breathlessness of discovery. Don't evaluate the response—it's part and parcel of your Yoga!

2. Did anything come up in your creation that helped you to better understand

    a. the asana itself?
    b. group dynamics?
    c. your personal creative process?
    d. how observing and being observed feels?
    e. responses and technical parts of the pose you'd like to take a deeper look at?

3. How do you think broader media portrayals of Hatha Yoga have influenced the practice in our cultural/historical milieu?

4. How do you think artistic portrayals of Hatha Yoga impact your practice?

Capping Poem:

I shake out the mat,

bits of sawdust and cedar twigs scatter in the slanting light,

homey glitter.

I work through my practice,

mindful of the mismatched socks of forward fold,

hiking up my bra straps after triangle,

and pushing my dog's slobbery face away from me

in Savasana

with a totally inappropriate giggle.

Somehow, I'm sure

I'll never make the cover

of any Hatha Yoga publication.

So much more satisfying to give in

to my pooch's Upward Facing Dog

transitioning elegantly to

Let's Go Play with the Ball Already Vinyasa.

Namaste, indeed.

Practice 23: Rising and Falling into the Still Point of Savasana

Perhaps you've noticed how often folks are sort of left hanging when it comes time for relaxation/corpse pose at the end of the practice. It's such a tough call. Do you "hold" participants with your voice and imagery or turn them totally loose to flounder around their still points with minimal way-showing?

This Inquiry will give you a practice that instructors and students alike can replicate quickly and easily. With new students, I walk everyone through the practice prior to doing it, so I can minimize my later verbal instructions. With more experienced groups who have worked with me for quite some time, I simply ask them to transition into Savasana and then, in seated meditation, mentally hold them in their Inquiries. Periodically, I ask "what came up for you in relaxation pose?" As a group we can then examine how the experience manifests across a broad range of folks.

I suggest you try this Inquiry without music and with music and see what happens!

Part One:

Ask students to draw their knees up to their chests in Reclined Child. Place a hand on each knee-cap. Draw the knees towards the chest on the exhale and allow the knees to move away on the inhale. Allow the student's natural breath to dictate the depth and speed of the flow. Continue for six to twelve breaths.

Part Two:

Feet come to the floor. Wiggle the pelvis until it is flat and even against the floor. Extend the legs, one at a time and then press the heels away from the sit-bones. Inhale, and then exhale and allow the legs to drop all their tension and fall into their most elongated, comfortable and natural lines.

Part Three:

Feel the belly and chest open with the breath. Following an inhale, encourage the rib cage and sternum lift a bit, allowing the shoulder blades to flatten against the mat. Arms tip out to the sides, palms up. Exhale and relax deeply.

Part Four:

Roll your head side to side very slowly and mindfully. Gradually decrease the rolling until you come to rest in stillness.

Part Five:

Place your concentration on the rise and fall of your breath around the heart or in your belly.

Part Six:

Each time you breathe in, imagine you are expanding, taking up space, filling above and all around you. Each time you breathe out, feel like you are sinking into the earth, being held with love and attention. Disengage from forcing the breath—allow it to find its best rhythm and depth. You are only observing, not controlling. As the breath slows and quiets, the sense of expansion and being held become subtler. Stay with both extremes, watching the changes taking place without struggle.

Part Seven:

You may at last find yourself in a place of stillness, inbreath and outbreath in equilibrium and almost not discernable, mind perfectly poised in that still point, body wholly relaxed and unguarded. If mind kicks back in, return to the practice of observing the expansion and sense of being held, always willing to simply begin again without self-judgement.

Part Eight:

When you are ready to release Savasana, first request your breath to deepen. Become conscious again of the expansion and sense of being held. Watch the effects of this transition carefully and with interest. After a few breaths, roll to your right side and take at least six deep and full breaths before coming to a seated meditation posture. Conclude this portion of your practice in a way that is right for you.

Part Nine:

When you are Inquiring about this technique, take some time to explore the following questions:

1. Are you typically comfortable with Relaxation pose? What have you observed about your experience of this asana in the past? Through time?

2. How did this practice affect

    a. your body?
    b. your breath?
    c. your Mind?
    d. your sense of intuition?
    e. your sense of joy?

Did this practice somehow both unify and transcend
these distinctions? Why do you think this
happened?

3.   This pose is called Corpse Pose in precise
     translations. Why? What does the name suggest
     to you and why might it be one of the most
     important asanas you explore? How do normal
     emotions like fear play into this asana?

4.   Can you truly verbalize what happens in the still
     point of Savasana? Explain.

5.   How is Savasana different from classical
     meditation techniques?

Capping Poem:

Inhale, exhale,

trail into each other,

white acrylic on white canvas,

while

the body easel floats,

confusing holding with being held,

and mind,

a cotton and linen and wrapped wood frame,

forgets again and again

how to grow,

pick

spin

and weave.

Intuitively, I could say more,

but joy

holds a finger to lips

Ssssshhhhhh.

Practice 24: Offering the Practice to Others

When you rise from Savasana, you may feel the need to do something more like meditate, intone a few Oms, and the like. This transition time highlights a basic human need for ritual and closure. Why not use this time to further your connection to others, and to invite yourself to transcend your practice as something that merely builds up your ego?

Part One:

After your time in Savasana, slowly enter a meditation posture, eyes closed.

Part Two:

Lift your arms to shoulder-height, palms to the ceiling. Notice how the gesture opens your heart.

Part Three:

Speaking aloud to your class (or making the intention out-loud in your own words if you are practicing by yourself)

"Send your practice to someone, someplace that could use it. Or simply allow it to return to the Mystery from which it unfolded."

Part Four:

Allow a few moments of silence, as you or others send forth the practice. Give the moment all your intention, all your goodwill, all your compassion.

Part Five:

In words or chant, intone the following mantra. If you wish, you can do it yourself or teach it to your class.

> *"Loka, samastha, sukino bhavantu*
>
> *OM Shanti, Shanti, Shanti"*

And then translate:

> *May all being enjoy peace, joy, love and light*
>
> *OM peace, peace, great peace*
>
> *Namaste, gentle people*

Close the practice with a bow to your students, palm to palm or to your practice space.

Part Six:

Take up your journal after class and consider how this Inquiry affected you. You might consider passing the questions out in print form or through an email/text message to your class and encourage them to bring their answers for the next practice day.

1. Imagine how a Yoga practice might feel if you simply jumped up after Savasana and broke into chatter with your friends. Compare that kind of ending with the Inquiry above. How does ending with intention and compassion affect the way you receive your practice? How does it affect the rest of your day?

2. Did you feel any resistance to ending the practice this way? If so, challenge yourself to create your own ritual closing! Share it with someone you love and trust. For instance, when teaching Christian Yoga, it

may be appropriate to end with a version of the Lord's Prayer.

3. What are the ramifications of giving your practice away? Be concrete.

4. Considering that many students must get into cars immediately after a class and navigate with an entirely different part of their brain, how can this practice ease this transition? What else does it provide your students? Try to think of at least three benefits this technique offers.

5. What other ways could you preserve and encourage a contemplative atmosphere in your class or home practice? Consider as many aspects of the environment (lighting, sound, music if any, and so on), as well as pre and post practice diet and hydration, media/cell phone/computer exposure and anything else you can recall. Share your insights with your class or begin to follow your own suggestions in your private practice. Observe and journal your observations over time.

Capping Poem:

Palm to palm I bow,

framing a dark space,

tiny and intimate cathedral of muscle, vein and bone.

Thumbs, oh so useful,

pressed against each other,

nestling toward the heart

instead of some activity.

This is Now,

all endings-beginning

held in holy tension

between two hands.

Practice 25: Rolling up the Mat

So how do you move off the mat and into your work day, your day of vacation or holding your new baby? Like the space between each asana, your entire waking existence can be broken down into transitions and thresholds. Beloved peace ambassador, Zen Buddhist monk and Nobel Peace Prize nominee Thich Nhat Hahn bows to each doorway he encounters through the day, because each space is liminal, opening to a fresh and new physical environment. This is just one way to awaken and greet the holy present moment.

By paying attention not only to the transitions between poses, but also the way you transition into your day or evening, you begin to live the message of your Hatha Yoga.

Let's give it a try with this simple Inquiry:

Part One:

After the closing of the class, mindfully step a little away from your mat. Palm to palm, bow to the sacred space you have created. Don't be afraid to use the religious tradition of your choice in a way that is right for you. Perhaps if you are Christian, you can ask God to bless the mat. As a Buddhist, it's like bowing to your meditation cushion, gratitude offered for the chance to practice wakefulness. You may also want to add words to roll your mat up with, like:

Thank you for holding my practice.

Thank you for holding all the parts of myself.

Thank you for serving as the doorway

into Union with the Divine.

OM Shanti, Shanti, Shanti

Part Two:

If you clean your mat each time, stay present to each motion, avoiding the urge to hurry.

Part Three:

Mindfully roll the mat. Stay present to each motion. Place the mat in its bag, strap or place in the studio or your home and again, press palm to palm and bow. You are not bowing *to* the mat, but rather, appreciating its presence the way an icon may be use—it is an intimate window into a different kind of consciousness.

Part Four:

Take the time to discuss the questions below with someone or jot down some answers in your journal:

1. How did you react to mindfully rolling up your mat on the level of your

    a. body?
    b. breath?
    c. mind?
    d. intuitive self?
    e. sense of joy?

2. What other liminal times call for the creation of a small ritual to move into a different kind of consciousness? For example, my husband and I always offer a prayer before every meal. What would you enjoy adding to your daily routine?

3. Does mindfully rolling up your mat add anything to the transition between class/practice and your daily activities? Explain.

4. Why does humankind use ritual in some fashion?
    What does ritual add to life?

5. If all your students practice this mat-mindfulness,
    how do you think it will affect your studio space?
    Your teaching style? Interactions between students?
    Try the inquiry and then journal about any changes
    you catch as it becomes routine.

Capping Poem:

How many doorways do I cross,

list in hand,

earbuds and hiking boots on,

keys jangling,

laughing about a Facebook joke?

How many times have I crossed from room to room,

forgotten where I came from

not noticing when I have arrived,

and usually forgetting why I was there?

How do I hold hellos and good-byes,

sleeping and awakening

births and deaths?

The same way?

About the Author

Kim Beyer holds a master's degree in comparative religion as well as graduate certificates in holistic healthcare, Hatha Yoga Therapy, Reiki, Spiritual Direction and Art for Healing. She is the author of over twenty books ranging from poetry to science fiction, and has taught Hatha Yoga, Qigong, meditation and adult education classes for over twenty-five years. She and her husband founded Family Wild, a company committed to deepening family connections through hunting, fishing and nature arts. Kim is an avid fiber artist, horse and dog lover, and enjoys playing her Native American flute.

*Join Kim's email group **The Daily View** and visit her blog and website at:*

www.vistaandcrossroads.com/blog